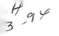

The Swiss Nature Doctor

The purpose of the books in this series is to awaken and kindle your interest in the many natural healing resources available all around you, and to demonstrate how simple, harmless remedies found in nature are often more effective than artificially created chemicals found in your local pharmacy, which may, in "curing" you, bring unpleasant and harmful side effects. By studying the advice given here, you will become acquainted with many hitherto secret, yet easily accessible, remedies from the Swiss folklore of healing which are only waiting to be discovered and put to good use.

The Swiss Nature Doctor's
LIBRARY OF NATURAL HEALTH

For information on this exciting series,
write to the Publisher

The Swiss Nature Doctor's Hints For a Healthier Liver

Dr. A. Vogel

Keats Publishing, Inc. New Canaan, Connecticut

The Swiss Nature Doctor's Hints for a Healthier Liver is not intended as medical advice. Its purpose is solely informational and educational. Please consult a medical or health professional should the need for one be indicated.

THE SWISS NATURE DOCTOR'S HINTS FOR A
HEALTHIER LIVER

ISBN: 0-87983-525-7

Published by Keats Publishing, Inc.
27 Pine Street (Box 876)
New Canaan, Connecticut 06840-0876

Table of Contents

The Liver—and What We Do to It

The liver is a marvel of divine technique. A single lobule of the liver, no larger than a pinhead, is a complete secreting unit in itself, and is made up of approximately 350,000 cells. When we consider that the liver contains a million of these lobules, we get some idea of the vastness of this chemical factory that filters and detoxifies no less than 600 liters of blood each day. Toxic substances reaching the liver via the portal vein from the intestinal tract are intercepted so that no harm comes to the body. Weighing about 1½ kilograms, or 3½ pounds, it is the largest gland in the human body.

It is clear that the liver is vital to our lives and our health, but it is abundantly true that we subject it to insults and injuries which impede its functioning in our service and threaten its very substance. The best known outright liver poison is alcohol, which causes the degenerative condition called cirrhosis, fatal to so many heavy drinkers; but chemicals in the air and water, additives and pesticide residues in food, the growing consumption of processed "foodlike" substances, excessive protein intake, food choices which strain the liver while failing to meet its nutritional needs—all these, and more, characterize the cruel and suicidal abuse to which we subject our livers.

When liver function is threatened, medical—drug—and surgical therapies are sometimes employed, but usually with limited success. Living and eating in a way which will avoid liver problems is the best approach, but it is not always possible to escape the toxins that surround us; and even the best of us will at times act short-sightedly or be unaware of proper diet. Therefore, we discuss here methods of improving impaired liver function drawn from nature's well-stocked armamentarium of remedies.

Blood Cleansing Cures

A general blood-cleansing cure, which is usually best undertaken in the spring (but can be done at other times) is one way of lightening the burden on the liver.

Wild plants such as dandelion, wild leek or bear's garlic (*Allium ursinum*), young nettles, yarrow, watercress and even the leaves of the pretty flowering nasturtiums are ideally suited for that purpose. Alfalfa, an extremely deep-rooted legume, is favored not only as a blood cleanser but also as a blood builder. Taken in conjunction with young nettles and oat grass, it is a particularly happy combination.

Obtaining the full value from a blood cleansing cure requires effective intestinal elimination. It is here that mucilaginous seeds such as psyllium and linseed come into their own. Soaked figs or prunes frequently achieve the same effect. Obstinate constipation does of course call for somewhat stronger-acting remedies. An effective and even pleasant measure is a laxative fruit paste: ten parts of soaked figs and prunes to one part (preferably powdered) senna pods are put through a blender or food mill, shaped into bars and rolled in dried coconut.

Detoxification with Rhubarb Leaves. If you have both a garden in which you grow the healthful and delicious rhubarb and a measure of privacy, you may don the costume of Adam (or Eve) and stretch yourself on a sunny flat roof or any place sheltered from inquisitive neighbors, and cover yourself from head to foot with rhubarb leaves. Remain under this verdant shelter for perhaps two hours or even longer. If the day is really hot, you will start to sweat copiously and may notice the odor of the eliminated toxins. If you repeat the cure twice or thrice, you will almost certainly feel much fresher and rejuvenated. The cure does not cost anything except the rhubarb leaves, which you would throw on the compost heap in any case, and a little time pleasantly and profitably spent.

Health Problems Associated with the Liver and How to Deal with Them

The earlier we become aware of any indisposition on the part of the liver, the better. Dislike of sweet things and fatty foods is one indication of this problem. A simple, well-proven remedy such as the juice of radishes, will be effective, and carrots, juiced or grated fine, even more so. All fat foods, as well as sweets, fruit and fruit juices, should be avoided. Here are some specific problems involved in liver malfunction and a brief description of remedies for them.

Infectious Liver and Gall Disorders. These usually manifest themselves in the form of a sick feeling and the vomiting of gall, which may be accompanied by diarrhea or even jaundice. Fasting is the quickest and most satisfactory cure. Continue it for a few days during which nothing is drunk except a glass of warm water in which a teaspoonful of white or yellow clay has been dissolved, fortified with a few drops of the homeopathic remedy Lachesis 12x. If bile is vomited, tea made from the horsetail or from dandelion roots and leaves will be very serviceable.

The Stomach and the Liver. There are stomach troubles which have their origin in a disordered liver. Quite naturally, therefore, we will consider the curative requirements of the liver when dealing with this kind of gastric infirmity: meals free from fruit and fat acids, but including plenty of readily digestible brown rice or such grains as millet, buckwheat and rye, should be accompanied by carrot juice and fresh salads—very definitely with a non-vinegar dressing, which can produce heartburn. A fundamental requirement for the cure of any gastric indisposition is of course thorough mastication and insalivation of the food.

Rheumatism, Arthritis and the Liver. Unless the liver's function has been undermined in some way, the toxins giving rise to rheumatism and arthritis could not accumulate. For this reason, a successful cure of these troubles is quite inconceivable without attention to the liver. No matter whether we employ the formic acid therapy, acupuncture or mud cures, they should be accompanied by measures designed to normalize liver function. Many a patient believes that the absence of liver pain is an indication that this organ plays no part on his illness. In this of course he is mistaken.

Eye Troubles and the Liver. Liver afflictions generally cause the circulation of the blood to become less vigorous, and when this happens, not only the various internal organs but also the eyes receive insufficient nutrients and the removal of metabolic wastes is slowed down. If this is allowed to go on for any length of time, the functioning of the eyes will suffer and clouding, inflammation and so on may occur. I have often observed that the successful treatment of circulatory disturbance has led to the disappearance of eye troubles—very much to the consternation of the eye specialists! Purification of the blood and stimulation of the liver should be included in any eye treatment.

Migraine and the Liver. The reader may question the assertion that there is an association between migraines and the liver, but the symptoms often accompanying these crippling headaches, such as nausea, sometimes with subnormal temperatures, and vomiting of gall, can most definitely be allocated to the liver. Some known triggering factors of migraines such as anger, excessive fatty or bad food and exhaustion also point to it. My father was a migraine sufferer, and I have inherited many of his genetic characteristics, so would not have been surprised if I had noticed a tendency to migraine in myself. My natural way of living seemed for a long time to overcome any such weakness, and I was grateful. Then at the age of 50 I contracted an infectious disease while traveling in the tropics, which affected my liver. As a consequence, I began to suffer from migraine attacks even more severe than my father had had; but as soon as the liver improved, the migraine became less frequent and violent, and later was not evoked except under extreme stress.

This shows both that a sensible way of life can keep hereditary weaknesses in check and that a liver dysfunction need not necessarily manifest itself in what are considered typical liver pains. The migraine sufferer would do well to consider the advice given later in this book for preserving and regaining liver health.

Cancer and the Liver. In the United States, I once conferred with a leading cancer researcher, who told me that not a single cancer patient had entered his institution who did not also have a disordered liver and pancreas; the observations of other researchers confirm this and suggest that cancer without liver and pancreas pathology is not possible.

Worry and other negative mental conditions can prove very harmful to the liver, which will in turn lead to an aggravation of the mental depression and a baneful repeating cycle. With a little determination, one can channel one's emotions, calm the troubled waters of the mind and establish some degree of serenity. Some warm-water applications, herbal poultices or herbal hip-baths favorably influence such states of mind by improving certain bodily functions, which in turn leads to an improved mental outlook.

Nutrition is of major importance in fundamental therapy of the liver, and aspects of this will be discussed in later sections of this booklet.

A diagnosis of cancer of the liver is a shattering experience for patients and their relatives, and hopelessness is a common reaction. Such a reaction, if understandable, is also destructive, as it robs the patient of the best chance of survival. An affirmative state of mind is no guarantee of cure of any condition, of course, but it is almost always a strong factor in the against-the-odds recoveries from "incurable" conditions which do occur. I am convinced that the fear of cancer and its wrong treatment are far greater killers than the disease itself.

Some natural healing principles which should be observed are:

Breathing, the intake of sufficient oxygen, is an absolute necessity in the case of malignant growths, as cancer cells are encouraged by a lack of oxygen. Regular deep-breathing exercises, if necessary under professional direction, should be part of every cancer therapy.

Nutrition, based on whole, natural foods, is an absolute necessity in the treatment of cancer. It must be realized that the body requires perfectly natural foods to retain or regain good health. Fried foods and most animal proteins are prohibited, yogurt and cottage cheese (but not milk, cream or butter) being allowed. Raw, organically grown vegetables are the mainstay of the liver patient's diet; spinach, leeks and carrots should appear almost every day. Detailed information appears later.

Natural remedies are abundantly available to the liver patient, and one plant known in the Swiss mountains and elsewhere has proved itself useful in cancer cases. The plant *Petasites officinalis* or butterbur, particularly in combination with mistletoe, has appeared to halt the progress of the disease and to reduce or eliminate pain. A calcium compound derived from nettles has also seen effective use. Papaya and linseed oil preparations are useful as well.

Fats, Oils and the Liver

Saturated and hydrogenated fats—those found in meat and butter, and in processed foods and oils—place a great strain on the liver, while unsaturated fats promote healthful metabolic activity; these are found in many plants, primarily seeds and nuts.

Wholesome Oils. The best oil for liver patients is walnut oil, but it is not easy to find. Cold-pressed sunflower and safflower and canola oils are also helpful. Sesame oil is another excellent oil, for it contains no less than 43% highly unsaturated fatty acids and some important mineral and protein compounds. Fresh linseed oil is also highly effective, and is currently experiencing a rise in popularity which is making it more familiar and available to consumers.

As discussed in the next section, protein derived from plants is easily and beneficially assimilated by liver patients, and one characteristic of many plant protein foods is their content of unsaturated fats and oils.

Plant Protein

For benefit to be obtained from proteins, they must be "raw." Excellent protein comes from both the plant and animal worlds, and both are wholesome and well tolerated by the patient, though the individual patient's idiosyncrasies must always be considered. We shall consider first the protein-containing plants suitable to a liver patient's diet, beginning with seeds and nuts. These should be well chewed and are best eaten in conjunction with whole-meal bread.

Sesame Seeds, a Priceless Food. Sesame is one of the most important foodstuffs in the orient, where protein-rich foods are scarce. Its tiny seeds are rich in minerals such as calcium, iron, phosphorus and silica, and contain an abundance of unsaturated fatty acids. They are essential both for the nerve cells and for the liver. They are good sprinkled on a whole-meal bread sandwich or mixed into muesli. Sesame seed paste, *tahini,* is a healthful sandwich spread, and an excellent substitute for peanut butter—which should be avoided by liver patients, as should the peanut itself, which is highly indigestible.

Walnuts. Fresh walnuts are excellent for liver patients. If possible, purchase new-harvest walnuts, for once they have become rancid and old, they constitute a danger to the weak liver. Walnut oil is well tolerated by the liver, and we may consider it not only as a food but as a remedy. Walnuts also stimulate intestinal function and so help relieve constipation.

Coconuts. These can be heartily recommended in their dried form, which can be mixed into breakfast food such as muesli. They must always be thoroughly masticated, and only the finely aromatic and untainted article should be served. Pastries are *not* made healthful or acceptable by the addition of coconut, however!

Sunflower Seeds. These are very good for the liver patient, but unfortunately do not keep well, so one should always be careful to buy them in their fresh state. The benefit is chiefly from the unsaturated fatty acids they contain and which enhance the digestive powers. The use of cold-pressed sunflower oil can also be recommended.

Pistachio Nuts. These are native to southern climates, where they are used in cases of liver trouble. They are a source of easily utilized fats and protein, and their green color indicates that they contain chlorophyll, another valuable constituent. Note that all nuts, including pistachios, should be eaten in their raw state, so that the fat and protein compounds remain unchanged.

Legumes and Soybeans. Legumes are rich in proteins but are not well tolerated by the liver patient and should not be among his protein source. (Hence the warning against peanuts, above; they are not in fact nuts but legumes.) Soy beans are the most digestible of the legumes, and soy flour or flakes may be used for variety in the diet. They contain lecithin, which is of value to the nerves, and ferments that stimulate the liver and aid digestion.

Animal Proteins

Total vegetarians will experience difficulty in meeting their protein requirements, and on the other hand, the "normal" mixed-diet adherent will also encounter troubles when he is ill, as he should forgo his favorite source of protein, meat.

Whole Milk and Yogurt. As a rule, fats and proteins are combined in our foods, and it is a good thing that this is so. Experience has taught me that it is not wise to separate fats and proteins in any one food when the welfare of the liver patient is concerned. Whole milk as a source of protein is for this reason an ideal article of diet, containing as it does, protein, fats and minerals. This happy combination is destroyed in the manufacture of butter, of which skimmed milk is a by-product. Neither is as wholesome and beneficial as the original whole milk, which, if it is consumed raw, is the best of all milk products.

Anyone who has difficulty in digesting it can take it sour or in the form of yogurt. Yogurt and sour milk have similar properties, are digested and assimilated better than milk, and improve intestinal function through their content of lactic acid bacilli, which can under some circumstances restore degenerated intestinal flora to normal. The practice of mixing fruit juices or conserves into yogurt cannot be encouraged, as lactic acid and fruit sugars are incompatible, leading to fermentation.

Cheese. Liver patients should abstain from fermented or "ripe" cheeses, as they may lead to considerable disturbances, especially if the patient also suffers from arthritis. Even the smallest quantities used as flavoring should be avoided.

Curd cheese, also known as white or cottage cheese, is without doubt the best fat and protein food from animal sources. Tomatoes go well with it for a healthful, delicious sandwich. It can accompany a vegetable meal in the form of a paste made by adding a little milk and flavored with garlic, grated horseradish, caraway seeds or vegetable juice.

If raw oil, as discussed earlier, does not agree with the patient, it can be made more digestible by mixing it with curd cheese.

Eggs. Though a rich source of protein, eggs should be eaten in moderation by those with liver problems, and preferably raw—if cooked at all, boiled no longer than two minutes. Boiled eggs, even as a garnish, should be avoided entirely, and eggs in any form are forbidden to arthritis patients.

Meat and Fish. In the treatment of liver patients, I have always had better results with those who abstained from meat. For one thing, the protein in which it is abundant is altered for the worse when it is cooked. As a concession to those who are in effect addicted to meat, fresh, first-quality veal or beef, grilled without fat, may be taken in small portions. Fatty meat and processed meats such as sausages are to be firmly avoided.

Critically ill patients cannot always do without liver, not so much as a food as a remedy. It must be given raw, which makes it quite unappealing. Liver extract may also be given, but either should be used for a limited period only.

Fish must be absolutely fresh, as ptomaine poisoning might prove fatal to the liver patient. They may be poached (in water only) or grilled without fat and served without butter or any similar dressing. An acceptable substitute for such dressings can be made with curd cheese, milk, cold-pressed oil and the juice of one lemon.

Grains for the Liver Patient

If it is necessary to eat whole-grain products in health, then it is even more necessary to avail ourselves of them when ill. White flour products constitute a starvation regime for the body and can under no circumstances be recommended, whether in the form of bread, buns, macaroni or biscuits. Let us be satisfied only with the best, nature-pure carbohydrates in their original state, in the form nature provides them. Then they will justify our expectation of finding even in cereals not only a food but a medicine.

Brown Rice. It is known that rice bran contains curative constituents that benefit the organism in general and the liver in particular. No wonder that diseases of the liver have never become a problem among rice-eating nations. Rice bran may be used as a supplement, but it is preferable to make whole, or brown, rice an article of diet.

Those who eat rice find that a large quantity is not required to still hunger for a long period, reducing the need for frequent meals, which rests the pancreas and therefore benefits the liver. Brown rice is more palatable than white rice, and is well worth the slight extra time it takes to prepare. It should be served two or three times a week at least.

Rye and Wheat. Rye is an excellent cereal and should be used more frequently. The outstanding effect of rye on the teeth is well known. If we do not want to cook whole rye, it can be used flaked, so long as it is fresh. Many rye crispbreads are wholesome and appetizing.

Wheat has most of the virtues of rye, and is slightly better assimilated, though rye is higher in mineral content and contains less starch. Wheat can be eaten in a variety of ways, cooked as a cereal, flaked or used in breads.

Oats. Oats are very beneficial to the nerves, and an excellent nerve tonic is prepared from the flowering oat plant. Diarrhea is favorably influenced by a mono-diet of oats; and, as might therefore be expected, oats should be used sparingly when constipation is a problem. Oats can be used in many ways, whole, flaked and as flour. Recent research has suggested that whole oats and oat bran lower levels of blood cholesterol, which would be another reason for using this versatile cereal.

Barley, Buckwheat, Millet and Corn. Barley is undeservedly unpopular, but can be useful in reducing internal heat, frequent in liver disorders, when infused like a tea and allowed to stand for some time. This barley water is popular in the tropics as a remedy for thirst and fevers.

Buckwheat, available in many areas under the name of *kasha,* is easily digested and can be prepared in a variety of ways. It is a very concentrated food, containing approximately 50% starch, 30-35% oil and 8% protein; it has a high content of silica, the great cleansing, eliminating and healing mineral salt, and thus offers many benefits to the liver.

Millet is also rich in silica, and can be served as a sweet or savory, baked in the oven and combined with salads and vegetables. It is highly nutritious and an excellent food for growing children.

The value of corn or maize is demonstrated by the American Indians, for whom it has been a staple diet. It can be eaten in cornmeal dishes or fresh from the cob.

The Best Way to Use Grains. Whole cereals retain their great power only as long as they retain the power to germinate. The aim of every kind of preparation should be to use all cereals as soon as possible after grinding, at which point the destructive process of oxidation begins. Every modern, progressive household should stock wheat, rye, barley, oats, buckwheat and millet as whole grains. They can be soaked overnight and put through a food mill the next day, or ground fresh whenever required. Sprouting grains is another healthful way of preparing them, and increases digestibility.

All genuine whole-meal breads, especially rye bread and the traditional Scandinavian crispbreads, are a boon for the liver. The liver patient must give special attention to the mastication of bread, so that the enzymes in saliva can act to release the nutrients. Avoid breads raised by chemical powders in favor of those employing natural yeasts or sourdough.

Wholesome Vegetables for the Liver

Vegetables are rich in mineral salts, enzymes, vitamins and a variety of other vital elements, as well as first-class protein. They possess both nourishing and healing qualities, and some vegetables have indeed very pronounced curative effects. However, many investigations have shown that the greatest nutritional and curative value is found only in foodstuffs that have been produced by organic methods, without chemical interference and in accordance with the biological laws governing soil and plant.

As a rule, raw vegetables have greater healing value than cooked ones, so that we should consume at least a substantial part of our green fare raw. When cooked, they should be steamed rather than boiled, and any cooking water remaining should be utilized in soups for its mineral content.

Vegetables of the brassica family such as cabbage, kale and brussels sprouts, which often promote flatulence when cooked, are better tolerated raw. To help heal the liver's infirmities, vegetables containing bitter substances, such as dandelion, chicory and endive, should frequently appear on the table, together with leeks, spinach and all kinds of leafy greens. Carrots are a "specific" for the sick liver, as are artichokes. Fennel is good, too, but legumes, as noted earlier, should be avoided.

Wild Plants. Growing where the nutrient balance of the soil is undisturbed, wild plants provide many healing benefits. One such plant is the nettle, rich in vitamin D, calcium and other mineral salts. Gather them young, cut them fine and add them to a raw vegetable salad or to soup after cooking. A nettle puree prepared like spinach and flavored with garlic is a tasty dish indeed! Dandelion leaves are among the first wild plant foods we can enjoy in early spring. They cleanse the liver and are a medicine rather than a food. Wild leek (bear's garlic, ramsons), whose leaves closely resemble those of lily-of-the-valley but whose pungent smell removes any confusion between the two, normalizes blood pressure, regenerates the blood vessels and is a good remedy for the infirmities of age. Collect the leaves and use them raw or steamed in the same way as nettles.

Spinach. If we cannot grow spinach ourselves, we should go to the trouble of finding a reliable source of supply of the organically grown produce. It is well worth the effort, for spinach contains plenty of iron and chlorophyll and is therefore an excellent blood medicine, which should be eaten raw as salad every day that it is in season. Cut fine, even the large, somewhat coarse leaves will be acceptable.

If spinach is to be cooked, it should be steamed in its own juice without the addition of fat. This can be done in special steaming utensils or in heavy-bottomed stainless steel pots. Spinach which has been soaked or cooked in water, especially after it has been cut up, is useless.

Spinach dumplings, made with raw spinach juice and wholemeal, make a pleasant change. A glass of spinach juice now and then enormously enriches our meals.

Radishes. Small quantities of radishes have been repeatedly recommended as a remedy for liver troubles. Let me emphasize that too many of them will harm rather than benefit us. The large black radish, *Raphanus sativus,* is one of the best liver medicines, if we consume it in small quantities, and will preserve the liver patient from gallstone colic and all sorts of digestive troubles.

Carrots. Disturbances in the function of the liver as well as actual liver diseases benefit enormously from raw carrots. With minor liver trouble, it will be found sufficient to fast for three or four days and take nothing but raw carrot juice. Cooked carrots are useless as a curative food, which means that we must take them either in the form of raw juices or finely grated in a salad—this is by far the best way.

Artichokes. Again and again I am surprised to what extent artichokes help in cases of liver disorders. A period of only two or three days is sufficient to furnish convincing proof of their efficacy as a liver remedy if they are eaten raw; along with the carrot, we may count them as one of the most curative dietetic articles we have at our disposal.

Raw artichokes are eaten in exactly the same way as the cooked ones; one leaf after another is peeled off to get at the tender part and the inside or "heart" of the artichoke. A dressing usually accompanies both steamed and raw artichokes, and there is no objection to this if it is made with creamy curd cheese, a good cold-pressed oil and lemon juice or whey concentrate. The lower part of the artichoke leaf is very tender and is as beneficial as the rest of the plant. If you insist on steamed artichokes, at least alternate them with raw, as these have much greater healing power. Artichokes should appear on the table at least two or three times a week, and if we want to enjoy their full benefits, we shall serve this valuable vegetable daily.

Cabbage. Grated raw and lightly seasoned, cabbage is an excellent source of vitamin C, calcium and other mineral salts and is therefore very beneficial for the liver. In some areas raw sauerkraut made from organically grown cabbage and fermented with lactic acid is available, and this is an excellent form of this useful vegetable.

Potatoes. Fried potatoes are taboo for the liver patient, who will find the steamed ones much more wholesome. Eaten with curd cheese and salads, they make a good and healthful meal. They must not be boiled in water but steamed, in order to retain most of their food value.

Although raw potatoes are anything but palatable, they are nevertheless a valued remedy for ulcers, rheumatism and arthritis as well as intestinal disturbances such as colitis and diarrhea resulting from a liver disorder. Raw potatoes are best taken finely grated in a vegetable soup or as juice, the taste of which can be wonderfully improved by the addition of carrot juice.

The Value of Vegetable Juices

The value of vegetable juices is becoming more and more widely recognized. Their specific effect is more pronounced than that of fruit juices, and, partly for this reason, they should not be used for long periods. The principle of wholeness demands that a sole-juice diet be used only temporarily, for it is only the whole plant that is capable of maintaining the physiological balance of our organism. This does not mean that we cannot take certain neutral juice such as carrot juice in small quantities quite regularly. We cannot live on juices alone, for we require not only easily assimilated nutrients but also indigestible material such as fiber as well to promote the proper functioning of the intestinal tract.

The Weekly Juice Day. Of great advantage is a weekly juice fast day, as it gives the body an opportunity to rest, giving every internal organ the chance to get rid of metabolic wastes and other accumulated impurities. The kidneys and liver derive great benefit from this measure. Nearly all vegetable juices are alkaline in reaction and have thus the advantage of balancing the pH of the system in our favor. Surplus alkaline elements unite with any free acids present, which changes metabolic toxins, uric and hydrochloric acid into new compounds which can be eliminated as salts in the urine.

For a vegetable juice day, we may use kale, cabbage, carrots, turnips and spinach—which must, of course, be grown organically. Of these juices we should take not more than a wineglassful (about 6 ounces) at one time, and not more than 4 to 6 glasses a day. For a systematic purification to eliminate uric acid and other urine-bound materials, we shall begin with a fortnightly juice day, which can later be repeated every week.

The Effect of Various Juices. Carrot juice benefits the liver, also the gall, provided not too much is taken. It increases the red coloring matter of the blood because of its concentrated nutrients, and is therefore an excellent blood medicine.

Spinach and turnip juices also increase the hemoglobin and benefit the liver in their raw state. Other juices, such as those of parsley, celeriac, watercress and radish, must be very carefully taken in doses determined by the body's tolerance. A wineglassful of radish juice may trigger colic when gallstones are present, while a teaspoonful helps to liquefy the gall and assist the function of the liver.

Raw juices must not be drunk like water, but held in the mouth and well mixed with saliva. Juices can be added to soups after cooking, if they cannot be taken raw.

Fruits, Berries and the Health of the Liver

Before discussing the role of fruit in the diet of the liver patient, we must point out that the use of chemical pesticides on fruit presents a health problem for everyone, well or ill. The utmost effort in obtaining fruit grown organically and without pesticides will be well repaid, and all other fruit should be thoroughly cleansed. At one time we spoke strongly against the peeling of fruit, as the best mineral salts are often found immediately below the skin, but today we must encourage it, for the benefit to be derived from the minerals is outweighed by the dangers of the contaminated skin.

That consideration aside, fruits present many problems for the liver patient, as they are comparatively difficult to digest and usually are acid. This is notably true of citrus fruits, except for grapefruit, for the bitter substances it contains are beneficial for the liver patient.

Mild apples may be enjoyed occasionally if they are thoroughly chewed and insalivated to neutralize the acid present. Pears can affect the liver and urinary organs, and need careful treatment. Sun- or air-dried pears may be enjoyed even by the liver patient if he pays attention to mastication and insalivation; but sulphured dried fruit must on no account be used.

Stone fruits should generally be avoided in cases of liver trouble, and if tried at all should be fully tree-ripened. Prunes, though, are quite wholesome and help to regulate the intestinal function; they are not usually sulphured, but this must be checked.

Grape sugar is valuable, and if grapes agree with the liver patient, it would be a pity not to use them. They must be conscientiously cleaned to remove any traces of spray, and skin and pits should be discarded. Raisins well chewed provide a pleasant and valuable supplementary food.

Fruit salads make demands upon the digestion, and are probably best avoided until the function of the liver has become normalized.

Berries. No other fruits contain so many concentrated healing elements as berries. Fortunately they grow well throughout the temperate zones. It is peculiar that our native berries cannot be found in the tropics, where they have mangoes and papayas, which can take the place of berries as they have similar properties of stimulating the liver and pancreas.

Proof of the healing effect and the wholesomeness of berries is supplied by those who suffer from liver and pancreatic disorders. No other local fruits are tolerated as well as the berries. Bilberries or blueberries can be eaten by the most severely ill liver patient, and what is more, they will actually help in restoring health.

It is somewhat of a puzzle that berries which taste sour are nevertheless alkaline in reaction. However, not everything that tastes acid remains chemically acid when it is ingested. Even those berries with a pronounced sour taste have in reality a surplus of alkaline substances, and therefore help in the de-acidification of the body. There is only one berry that has an acid surplus, the cranberry.

Berry juices are a therapeutic of the first order, although we must never forget that the whole fruit is better and more valuable than the juice alone. As mentioned, bilberries or blueberries and their juices are excellent for the liver. So are fully ripe black-berries and black currants.

The Question of Sweeteners

Our consumption of sweets far exceeds any requirement, and at the same time their quality is in general not high. The amounts of sweets consumed at holidays alone are a real danger to health. Gastric and liver troubles as well as gallbladder problems frequently occur as the result of such excesses, and the combination of white flour, white sugar and inferior, heated fats which make up many festive "treats" is in itself harmful. If our daily food should consist of natural whole foods, it is no less important that our desire for sweets should be met with natural whole food.

Honey—the Best Sweetening Agent. Containing 40% dextrose and 35% levulose, honey is a highly concentrated source of energy. Dextrose need not be digested but can be absorbed straight away, quickly renewing strength. Levulose is assimilated slowly, supplementing the quick-acting dextrose with its sustained-release effect. Honey also contains important trace elements such as copper, manganese, and iron in an easily assimilated form; and its varied vitamin content is proportioned in accordance with the body's needs. It should be used in preference to other sugars, and is particularly useful for people with weak digestions and disturbed pancreatic function. Because of its concentration, honey should not be taken in excess.

Natural Grape Sugar and Other Fruit Sweeteners. Grape sugar is also an excellent, nutritious sweetener, and raisins and sultanas provide a healthful way of satisfying a desire for sweets. They must, of course, be sun-dried and not sulphured. In utilizing these dried grapes for sweetening purposes, soak them in water overnight and put them through a food mill or blender.

Artificial grape sugar, made from potato or cornstarch, has the same chemical formula as the natural product, but lacks the nutrient value of the real thing, and should be avoided.

Another fruit sugar with some value is brown sugar—if and only if it consists of nothing but the condensed and crystallized juice of the sugar cane. Its mineral content is 80% alkaline, 20% acid, which is helpful.

As mentioned in the section on fruit, dried pears can be beneficial for the liver patient so long as they are prepared completely naturally; they can satisfy any desire for sweets. They contain iron and copper in organic form, which have important benefits for the blood.

Healthy Techniques of Eating and Drinking

Hurried eating is definitely harmful. If we feel we are keyed up and tense before a meal, we should sit in an armchair and relax. There must be peace at the table, so that we can give attention to thorough mastication and insalivation and to slow eating. On no account should food be washed down with drinks.

More or less the same applies to drinking. It is best to drink after meals, so that we have no opportunity to reach for the glass. All drinks, no matter whether cold or warm, and especially fruit and vegetable juices, must be as well insalivated as solid food.

These are the golden rules applicable to eating and drinking, and should be followed faithfully.

Dr. Alfred Vogel—"The Nature Doctor" in Person

For most of this century, Dr. Alfred Vogel has been learning the secrets of natural healing and the curative powers of herbs, and for almost as long has shared that knowledge with patients at the clinic he ran for many years and with countless readers of his many books. Born in 1902 near Basel, Switzerland he eagerly absorbed herbal lore from his grandparents and parents, eventually becoming familiar with the whole body of European empirical folk medicine. In later years he traveled to the remotest parts of the world and absorbed the curative lore of tribal peoples in Africa, Asia, Australia and the Americas. His stay with the Sioux Indians in South Dakota was among the most informative and inspiring of his many tribal encounters, and his great interest in all methods of natural healing led him to the study and use of homeopathic treatments as well.

In his worldwide lectures and the newsletter he has published for more than sixty years, Dr. Vogel has brought his experience and wisdom to many thousands, but it is his books, beginning as far back as 1925, that have carried that wisdom, and a legion of practical instructions for the full range of health problems, to a myriad of readers in many countries. His most famous work is *Der kleine Doktor*, published in English as *The Nature Doctor* and translated into eleven languages. Completely revised and enlarged, with exciting new information, this enduring classic of natural healing is the basis of this series of short guides to abundant health.

Dr. Vogel's decades of research and discovery have brought him professional recognition in many countries as well as the gratitude of those he has helped; he was granted an honorary doctorate in medical botany by the University of California at Los Angeles in 1952, and in 1982 was awarded the coveted Priessnitz Medal at the annual Congress of German Nature Cure Practitioners.

Though nearly ninety, Dr. Vogel still puts in a five-hour work day and attends many professional meetings and conferences, often finding that the latest research "discovers" what he has been practicing for seven decades—and what folk medicine has known for centuries. "Only nature can heal and cure," Dr. Vogel is fond of observing, adding the corollary that "we can help and support nature and its laws that make a cure possible." This has been the basis of his lifelong work.

Bioforce: Founding and Growth. In 1963 Dr. Vogel founded Bioforce, now one of the major manufacturers of herbal extracts, homeopathic medicines, specialty health foods and biological cosmetics. The original production facility was located in the small farming community of Roggwil, and new ones have also been sited to allow for growth and collection of the most helpful herbs at their freshest. Experienced collectors know the best times to gather wild herbs for maximum therapeutic potency, and production employs biological methods rather than chemical or mechanical wherever possible.

Dr. Vogel is responsible for the formulations of all Bioforce products, and draws on the full range of his experience, studies and travels to assure their safety and effectiveness. Some of the most popular remedies are combinations of herbs described in booklets in this series, such as Echinaforce, Dormeasan, Crataegisan, Boldocynara, Usneasan and Symphosan, which may be obtained from herbalists or in health stores in the thirty countries Bioforce exports to.

Information on specific remedies or on Bioforce products in general may be had from the main office:

Bioforce AG
CH-9325 Roggwil/TG
SWITZERLAND

or from regional headquarters:

Bioforce of America Ltd.
PO Box 507
Kinderhook, NY 12106
USA

A. Vogel of Switzerland
111 Gorham Street
Newmarket, ON L3Y 7V1
CANADA

Bioforce UK Ltd
South Nelson Industrial Estate
Cramlington
Northumberland NE23 9HL
UNITED KINGDOM

Bioforce Australia
PO Box 890
Eltham 3095, Victoria
AUSTRALIA

Bioforce Singapore Pte. Ltd.
327 River Valley Road 03-02
Yong An Park
SINGAPORE 0923

The Swiss Nature Doctor

For more than 60 years, Dr. Alfred Vogel, a third-generation herbalist, has been gathering the lifesaving lore of folk medicine from his native Switzerland and from the far reaches of the world, sharing his discoveries with the patients at the clinic he conducted for many years and with the millions of readers of his classic compendium, *The Nature Doctor.*

Now, distilled from the 1990 edition of this international bestseller, this series presents essential information and advice on a wide range of important areas of your health.

Ready now

HOME TREATMENT OF COMMON AILMENTS
SECRETS OF THERAPEUTIC HERBS
GUIDE TO A HEALTHIER HEART AND CIRCULATORY SYSTEM
RECOMMENDED FOODS FOR HEALTH AND VITALITY
HEALTHFUL ADVICE ON NATURAL DIET
BOOK OF 12 HEALTH-RESTORING TREATMENTS
HINTS FOR A HEALTHIER LIVER
LIVING THE ACTIVE LIFE AT AGE 90
BOOK OF 14 AMAZING HERBAL MEDICINES

Keats Publishing, Inc.
27 Pine Street
New Canaan, Connecticut 06840

Printed in U.S.A.
Cover design: Irving Bernstein

ISBN 0-87983-525-7

50295 >

EAN

9 780879 835255